The Culture Cure Mastermind Guide for Healthcare Transformation

The Culture Cure Mastermind Guide for Healthcare Transformation

...

Pamela M Tripp MEd, MSOM

Copyright © 2017 Pamela M Tripp MEd, MSOM
All rights reserved.
ISBN-13: 9781975811167
ISBN-10: 197581116X

The Eagle Creed

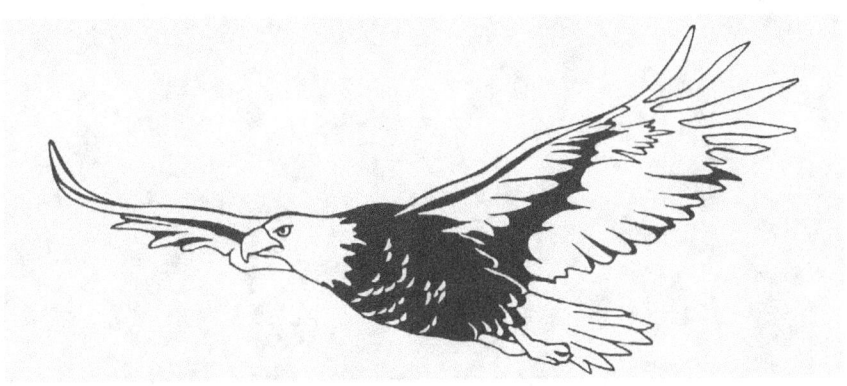

"What you settle for stays with you. Why settle for average when you can be phenomenal? Why live in a chicken coup when you can soar like an eagle? You are the gatekeeper of your destiny. Shut the door to ordinary and open your life to extraordinary."

Contents

Introduction · ix
   Mastermind Group Facilitation Tips · · · · · · · · · · · · · · · · · · · xii
   The Power of a Mastermind Group · xv
   Additional Resources · xvii

Module 1: Ch 1-2 — Valuing People · 1
   Reading Notes: Chapters 1-2 · 1
   Mastermind Discussion Guide Module 1 · · · · · · · · · · · · · · · · · 4
   Self-Reflection & Action Module 1 · 9

Module 2: Ch 3-4 — Engaging the Vision · · · · · · · · · · · · · · · · · · 13
   Reading Notes: Chapters 3-4 · 13
   Mastermind Discussion Guide Module 2 · · · · · · · · · · · · · · · · · 16
   Self-Reflection & Action Module 2 · 21

Module 3: Ch 5 — Fostering Leadership · · · · · · · · · · · · · · · · · · · 25
   Reading Notes: Chapter 5 · 25
   Mastermind Discussion Guide Module 3 · · · · · · · · · · · · · · · · · 28
   Self-Reflection & Action Module 3 · 34

Module 4: Ch 6 — Engage Empathy · 37
   Reading Notes: Chapter 6 · 37
   Mastermind Discussion Guide Module 4 · · · · · · · · · · · · · · · · · 40
   Self-Reflection & Action Module 4 · 45

Module 5: Ch 7 — Taking Ownership · 49
    Reading Notes: Chapter 7 · 49
    Mastermind Discussion Guide Module 5 · · · · · · · · · · · · · · · · · · · 52
    Self-Reflection & Action Module 5 · 58

Module 6: Ch 8 — Developing Strengths · 61
    Reading Notes: Chapter 8 · 61
    Mastermind Discussion Guide Module 6 · · · · · · · · · · · · · · · · · · · 64
    Self-Reflection & Action Module 6 · 70

Module 7: Ch 9 — Equipping Colleagues · 73
    Reading Notes: Chapter 9 · 73
    Mastermind Discussion Guide Module 7 · · · · · · · · · · · · · · · · · · · 76
    Self-Reflection & Action Module 7 · 81

Module 8: Ch 10 — Unleashing Empowerment · · · · · · · · · · · · · · · · · · · 85
    Reading Notes: Chapter 10 · 85
    Mastermind Discussion Guide Module 8 · · · · · · · · · · · · · · · · · · · 88
    Self-Reflection & Action Module 8 · 93

Module 9: Ch 11 — Driving Momentum · 97
    Reading Notes: Chapter 11 · 97
    Mastermind Discussion Guide Module 9 · · · · · · · · · · · · · · · · · · · 100
    Self-Reflection & Action Module 9 · 104

Module 10: Ch 12 — Hardwiring Success · 107
    Reading Notes: Chapter 12 · 107
    Mastermind Discussion Guide Module 10 · · · · · · · · · · · · · · · · · · 110
    Self-Reflection & Action Module 10 · 115

About the Author · 119
Corporate Transcendence · 121

Introduction

• • •

The Culture Cure Mastermind Group (MMG) is a powerful way to support deeper thought, self-reflection, and real world application of the foundational principles covered in the book, *The Culture Cure: Transforming the Modern Healthcare System* by Pamela M. Tripp. The MMG process will allow a group of 2 or more to share perspectives around what is being communicated and learned from each chapter in the book.

It is through an open dialogue of thoughts and shared ideas, that new perspectives, actions, behaviors are formed. This guide format is user friendly and allows a beginner, novice, or expert to be comfortable facilitating the MMG.

FACILITATOR ROLE

It is important to understand that the facilitator's role is not one of a teacher. The facilitator's purpose is to support the navigation of the topics and questions discussed among the MMG participants. To support new perspectives and thoughts, so that a third innovative and creative mind of thinking is gained among the participants.

WHAT TO EXPECT

There are 10 modules to the Mastermind Guide that can be divided into 10 weeks, of one hour sessions. The first MMG Module begins with Chapters

1 and 2 in the book. More or less time may be adjusted for a Mastermind session based on desires of participants. An important point to consider is that exploration of shared perspectives is needed for meaningful self reflection and new thought formation. This will greatly enhance the MMG experience. Participants are asked to read the corresponding chapter prior to a specific week's MMG. The MMG begins with a discussion around the most important thoughts revealed to the reader based on each chapter. Participants are encouraged to underline sentences and make reading notes that resonate with them.

There is designated space for note taking within the MMG for each Module under Reading Notes, that will be useful during MMG participation.

Questions within the MMG guidebook are designed to stimulate thought and communication. Questions and responses are to be shared openly in a safe climate of mutual value for each member's participation.

If there is a larger MMG, it may be more intimate to divide into groups and answer the participants' questions among 2-4 participants with a chosen spokesperson, then come back to the whole group for additional collective discussion.

After the questions are answered, the MMG participants have the opportunity to take a more personal self-reflection time under the section titled: Self-Reflection & Action. Self-reflection is the pathway to having your thinking come to life in your work.

Work through the the 4 I's to initiate self-reflection and future action. Allow this time to investigate your personal attitude and action. Ask "What am I going to do to embody these concepts and inspire others? What can I take action on, myself, as an individual?"

How can I....

- ❏ Be INSPIRED by the content that I have learned? What are ways that I can inspire and encourage people with these ideas?
- ❏ INFLUENCE others in my behaviors based on my new awareness? How can I personally use my influence to reflect and draw these behaviors out in others?

- ❏ INNOVATE among my colleagues to sustain my new learning? How can my colleagues and I bring innovation with this into our workplace?
- ❏ IMPACT my overall work environment based on my learning experience?

Do not allow participants to move to the action steps without adequate time for self-reflection and processing of module material. Self-reflection is key to learning.

Mastermind Group Facilitation Tips

PARTICIPANTS: Create a dynamic MMG by inviting participants from the frontline to executive leadership, volunteers, or even the general public. Anyone who has an interest in better understanding healthcare and who wants to gain insight on foundational principles needed to make positive culture transformation in the healthcare industry.

ROUND TABLE SEATING: Try to use round table seating when possible to allow people to face each other and better foster discussion. A more relaxed environment with comfortable seating may be suitable for small groups. Avoid classroom seating because it minimizes interaction.

BREAK INTO SMALL GROUPS: To maximize the involvement of every member with larger groups, remember to break up into groups of 2-4 people to answer the discussion questions. Have each smaller group choose someone to share their ideas with the whole group.

FIND THEMES & TRENDS: Gather the ideas from all the groups onto a whiteboard or poster board. Try to find a theme or trend among responses. Some groups like to use sticky notes and group similar responses together. Others use different color markers and circle recurring themes or contrasting experiences.

A SPECIAL TOUCH: Offering drinks or light refreshments can provide an extra touch that encourages people to participate and engage the group openly.

HELPFUL TOOLS:

- ❏ White Board or Poster Board
- ❏ Multi-Color Markers
- ❏ Sticky Notes
- ❏ Pens & Pencils
- ❏ Timer or Stopwatch

CHANGE UP PARTNERS: A great MMG discussion comes from unexpected conversation. Humans are creatures of habit, and often will sit with the same friend every week. Get creative to make new groups and spark fresh discussions among different participants.

An easy way to create unexpected groups is to COUNT OFF. See how many groups you would need to make to keep them at approximate 3-5 participants each, and count off up to that number going around the room. If you need 5 groups, start at one end of the room or table and give each person a number 1-5. Then have everyone switch up to sit with their group number. Even if you only need 3 groups, this method will increase the variety and add lots of energy to the discussion.

TEACH EACH OTHER: In a mastermind group, everyone is there to share with each other. We are learning from one another's experiences, wrestling with their ideas, and finding wisdom through reflection. Be sure to listen closely to all participants. Many times there is not an obvious answer without deeper thought and more self-reflection!

SELF-REFLECTION IS KEY: Every MMG participant should look for personal time to be thinking long beyond the hour. On many occasions, the power of a MMG comes to life in the hours and days after the meeting is over, so encourage self-reflection at every opportunity.

When facilitating or participating in a mastermind group, you only need to remember two things:

1. **Every participant has answers.** Positions and titles are left at the door when it comes time to innovate. Transformational ideas come from the most unexpected places, so be curious and take the time to draw every member into discussions. What they have to share with the group may surprise you.
2. **A Facilitators number one job is to create safety.** An important aspect of a facilitator is to create an environment where people feel safe to bring their gifts, share their ideas, and dare to begin the exciting, vulnerable work of hoping for change. Create an environment of learning and growth.

This guide is divided into 10 modules, designed to guide you and a group of colleagues through the core culture elements that can transform any healthcare organization from *The Culture Cure: Transforming the Modern Healthcare System*. Use this *Mastermind Guide*, to help you guide the group through the study and discussion of *The Culture Cure*, and invite every member to get a copy of *The Culture Cure Mastermind Guide*.

Whether you're in an authority role or not, you can step up and encourage others to begin transforming their environment by using this simple guide. Take the time to read through each module's talking points before each Mastermind meetup, and reflect on your own ideas so that you can be ready to engage the participants when they arrive. Each participant can use a copy of *The Culture Cure Mastermind Guide*, to participate in the discussion, and have helpful reflection and takeaways every week.

Invite your friends and colleagues to read *The Culture Cure* along with you, but know that even if you're the only one reading the whole book, great things will happen for everyone who attends and participates in the discussion and reflection.

Get creative in your meeting times, use the opportunity to be more connected to one another, and share ideas around these concepts. The first, most difficult battle we face in transforming our healthcare system is that of connecting and energizing the *people* in our industry. We need to get connected to one another, our strengths, and the transformational concepts discussed in this *Mastermind Guide*.

You're on the frontlines of healthcare transformation. Congratulations! Just by beginning your mastermind group, you are making a difference!

The Power of a Mastermind Group

This guide is designed to help you to engage a mastermind group around the specific principles of healthcare transformation delivered in *The Culture Cure: Transforming the Modern Healthcare System*. There has been a long, powerful tradition of mastermind groups in history. In fact, Napoleon Hill in 1920's is credited as one of the first people to use the term "Mastermind."

If you've ever been part of a mastermind group before, you know that incredible things happen when you get people in a room, and create the space to tackle important problems, discuss ideas, and take action together.

Some mastermind groups are designed very intentionally, perhaps bringing together the entire management team at your organization, or including everyone from a particular department. Other masterminds are casual, made up of a mishmash of friends who care about a topic, and make time to regularly get together and share a meal or cup of coffee, to brainstorm and connect with one another.

Pamela M Tripp MEd, MSOM

Mastermind Group: The Big Payoff

Mastermind sessions are an opportunity to bring people together who may work at the same organization, but do not have time to build a team relationship, and interact on a more personal basis. Understanding more about each other is key to developing winning teams with the mission of working together for excellent patient care. Mastermind groups are foundational in breaking down silos among individuals and departments. Synergy is built upon the relationship many times created through the MMG experience.

To deliver multidisciplinary, integrated WHOLE health, this requires a new type of leadership thinking. Leaders must embrace ways to build collaboration among all colleagues among all levels of the organization.

Understanding culture transformation beginning with *The Culture Cure* book and *Mastermind Guide*, is an excellent way to break ground in your organization, and begin to cultivate the work environment to become a high reliable and significant modern healthcare system.

Enjoy your journey!

ADDITIONAL RESOURCES

FURTHER WRITING BY PAMELA M. TRIPP:
For free resources and to be notified of Pamela's upcoming books, visit her author website, www.PamelaTripp.com. There you will be able to read her articles and keep up with her activities. For access to exclusive free culture assessment and leadership support resources, register for her email list. Subscribers receive exclusive content that can help executive and frontline healthcare leaders begin turning the tide to a more positive work environment.

CORPORATE TRANSCENDENCE™:
To learn more about the Corporate Transcendence™ culture transformation curriculum, visit www.CorporateTranscendence.com. If you are interested in transforming your healthcare organization with an evidenced based blueprint, or would like to invite Pamela M. Tripp to speak for your group, organization, or conference visit the Corporate Transcendence website to contact her team.

THE CULTURE CURE: TRANSFORMING THE MODERN HEALTHCARE SYSTEM.

Paperback: ISBN 978-1533661302
Ebook: ASIN: B01MEEUQ2M
Audiobook: ASIN: B01MZG4VDZ

COMPLIMENTARY CULTURE ASSESSMENT:

www.PamelaTripp.com/Free-Work-Culture-Assessment

CONNECT ON SOCIAL MEDIA:

Facebook: Facebook.com/OfficialPamelaTripp
            Facebook.com/CorporateTranscendence
            Facebook.com/TheCultureCure

LinkedIn: LinkedIn.com/in/PamelaTripp

MODULE 1

Valuing People

• • •

When we intentionally open our minds and hearts to appreciate our colleagues and the patients we serve, it creates a golden thread that runs through the organization. This positive relationship connection creates a solid foundation for cultural excellence.

~ Pamela Tripp

Reading Notes: Chapters 1-2

Use the following pages to take notes while you read. Pay special attention to concepts you think would be interesting to discuss at your MMG meeting:

_____
_____
_____
_____
_____
_____
_____
_____
_____
_____
_____
_____

The Culture Cure Mastermind Guide for Healthcare Transformation

നു
MASTERMIND DISCUSSION GUIDE
Module 1: Valuing People
Chapters 1-2

DISCUSSION TOPIC #1:
Innovation comes from the front line.

In chapter 2 of *The Culture Cure*, research shows that innovation and effective problem solving comes from the individuals doing that particular work. We often call these colleagues the front line. Lasting solutions require the ideas and input from the people doing work at every level. Involving frontline staff in performance, process, and systems improvement is key for creating a transcendent healthcare culture.

I. In your organization, how do you rally or engage the front line in performance improvement?

_____

II. How does your organization tap into innovative and creative ideas from all team members?

_____

III. What have you experienced in your organization by having frontline staff provide ideas for improving processes and services, and how can this be encouraged in your organization?

_____
_____
_____
_____
_____
_____

IDEA STARTERS:

A. Have you considered setting up **"Bright Idea Boxes?"** Place feedback boxes in common areas and encourage all levels of staff to share ideas as they come to them. Reward and acknowledge submissions in a timely manner to encourage increasing participation.

B. Are you **building teams with frontline employees**, or do you have management-only teams that are missing out on their ideas altogether? Teamwork makes the dream work. Avoid making decisions in a silo, without the insight of people who are doing the work every day.

REMEMBER: People are the experts on what they do every day!

DISCUSSION TOPIC #2:
The practice of "valuing" people.

In chapter 2, *The Culture Cure* talks about the concept of "valuing others," and defines it as "intentionally opening our minds and hearts to appreciate our colleagues and the patients we serve."

Taking time at the beginning of meetings to invite the team to acknowledge the excellence, attitude, and hard work of a colleague is *valuing* them. Making it a priority to give credit and praise to people who are doing the important daily work changes the energy on the team.

I. Could you see yourself providing a time for *Valuing* at the beginning of team meetings, perhaps even introducing it as the new way to start things off?

_____
_____
_____
_____
_____
_____

II. What are ways your organization can practice the value of *valuing* people?

_____
_____
_____
_____
_____
_____
_____

III. What practices are in place that make it easy to recognize and validate the work that people are doing well?

_____
_____
_____
_____
_____
_____
_____

IDEA STARTERS:

A. **Instant Reward and Recognition Opportunities.** If someone notices a colleague doing something outstanding, are there systems in place where they can be "written up" for their positive behavior? Connecting your recognition awards to your organization's core values is a great way to reward colleagues and to emphasize the behaviors associated with the values. Having an instant reward like a candy bar creates a powerful pattern of valuing and positive reinforcement for great service.

Take it to the next level by having everyone who gets recognized during the month entered into a drawing for a gift card or something more substantial.

B. **A Really Big Trophy.** Healthcare organizations work very hard to get everyone involved in Best Practices development and Patient Experience Satisfaction score improvements. Because patient satisfaction scores are so important, consider a Really Big Trophy (RBT) that lives right out front, in the department with the highest score. Every few months, move the trophy to whichever department has the highest score at the time. Team members get their pictures taken with the trophy, and the whole department celebrates!

Every day the RBT stands as a reminder that victory requires a team, and that every colleague is part of leading a department or organization to excellence.

SELF-REFLECTION & ACTION
Module 1: Valuing People
Chapters 1-2

It's all about my personal attitude and action. What am I going to do to embody and inspire others as an individual?

Four I's Model of Self-Reflection

How can I....

❑ How can I be INSPIRED by the content that I have learned? What are ways that my colleagues and I can inspire and encourage people with these ideas?

_____
_____
_____
_____
_____

❑ How can I INFLUENCE others in my behaviors based on my new awareness? How can I personally use my influence to reflect and draw these behaviors out in others?

_____
_____
_____
_____
_____

❏ How can I INNOVATE among my colleagues to sustain my new learning? How can my colleagues and I bring innovation with valuing into our workplace?

_____
_____
_____
_____
_____

❏ How can I IMPACT my overall work environment based on my learning experience?

_____
_____
_____
_____
_____

FACILITATOR'S NOTE: Do not allow participants to move to the action steps without adequate time for self-reflection and processing of module material. Self-reflection is key to learning.

Take Action

Who do you know who is a great example of *valuing* people?

_____

Will you find a chance to tell them you've noticed them, and appreciate the way they value others this week? (Circle Yes/No)

YES   NO

What is *one thing* you can do this week to engage the practice of valuing people and make valuing others a daily part of your culture at work?

_____
_____
_____
_____
_____
_____
_____
_____
_____
_____
_____
_____

MODULE 2

Engaging the Vision

• • •

Vision must develop legs and walk in daily operations to become reality.

~ Pamela Tripp

Reading Notes: Chapters 3-4

Use the following pages to take notes while you read. Pay special attention to concepts you think would be interesting to discuss at your MMG meeting:

_____
_____
_____
_____
_____
_____
_____
_____
_____
_____
_____
_____
_____
_____
_____
_____
_____

Pamela M Tripp MEd, MSOM

The Culture Cure Mastermind Guide for Healthcare Transformation

MASTERMIND DISCUSSION GUIDE
Module 2: Engaging the Vision
Chapters 3-4

DISCUSSION TOPIC #1:
Vision belongs to every person on the team.

Vision is *everything*. In chapter 4 of *The Culture Cure*, vision is described as "the overarching goals and aerial view of the future. It's not only who we are, but also who we are trying to become." You cannot visualize if your mind's eye cannot see.

I. What is the vision statement of your organization?
_____
_____
_____
_____
_____
_____
_____

II. How well do you understand what that vision means?
_____
_____
_____
_____
_____
_____
_____

III. Through colleague and corporate vision sharing, where do you see the organization 3-5 years down the road?
_____
_____
_____
_____
_____
_____
_____

IV. For the vision to become reality, that means every colleague must personally own the vision. Do you see this happening in your organization?
_____
_____
_____
_____
_____
_____
_____

V. Where do you see areas of disconnection between colleagues and the organization's vision?
_____
_____
_____
_____
_____
_____
_____

VI. What would happen if every member of the organization, at every level, grasped and understood where the vision is trying to lead? Would this impact daily priorities? Would it influence decision making? Would it keep energy focused on the most important things?

_____
_____
_____
_____
_____
_____
_____

IDEA STARTERS:

A. Is the organization's mission and vision visible throughout all areas and departments? Make it easy to keep the vision in mind by **Printing and Displaying the Vision** where everyone can see it. Read it at team meetings and remind colleagues of the greater meaning behind their daily work. Add pictures of colleagues to the vision statement on the wall!

B. Use your organization's Mission and **Vision Words** when you praise and acknowledge the efforts of others. If, for example, your vision talks of patient care excellence; commend people for "living out our vision for excellence in patient care," rather than simply saying "thanks for doing your job." People love making a positive difference with organizations that want to make a difference.

REMEMBER: Vision brings energy and hope. Don't go without it!

DISCUSSION TOPIC #2:
How do we translate the vision into daily action?

As big as vision may be, it cannot come to life if it stays locked in the executive board room. The vision has to come to life at every level for every colleague and stakeholder in the organization.

I. What do you need to do in your role in order for the vision to come to life?
_____
_____
_____
_____
_____
_____
_____

II. What challenges on a daily basis keep the vision from becoming reality?
_____
_____
_____
_____
_____
_____
_____

III. What weekly action steps would allow the vision to come to life?
_____
_____
_____
_____
_____
_____
_____

IV. How can the organization's mission and vision be positively aligned with a colleague's personal aspiration for the organization?

___

II. IDEA STARTERS:

A. Draft **Job-Specific Vision Statements**. Take the company vision and re-write it in terms of your specific job. Answer the question "What does great look like in your job?" How does that align with the vision of the organization?

B. **Prompting through Questions**. Get in the habit of asking yourself at the beginning of every work day "what am I doing today to move our organization toward our vision?" Perhaps post this question in your work area as a constant reminder.

FACT: The loftier your vision is, the more important everything becomes.

SELF-REFLECTION & ACTION
MODULE 2: ENGAGING THE VISION
CHAPTERS 3-4

It's all about my personal attitude and action. What am I going to do to embody and inspire others?

FOUR I'S MODEL OF SELF-REFLECTION

How can I....

❑ How can I be INSPIRED by the content that I have learned? What are ways that my colleagues and I can inspire and encourage people with these ideas?

_____
_____
_____
_____
_____
_____
_____

❑ How can I INFLUENCE others in my behaviors based on my new awareness? How can I personally use my influence to reflect and draw these behaviors out in others?

_____
_____
_____
_____
_____
_____
_____

❏ How can I INNOVATE among my colleagues to sustain my new learning? How can we bring innovation with this into our workplace?

_____
_____
_____
_____
_____
_____
_____

❏ How can I IMPACT my overall work environment based on my learning experience?

_____
_____
_____
_____
_____
_____
_____

FACILITATOR'S NOTE: Do not allow participants to move to the action steps without adequate time for self-reflection and processing of module material. Self-reflection is key to learning.

Take Action

Who do you know who is a great example of *knowing* and *living the vision*?

_____

Will you find a chance to tell them you've noticed them, and appreciate the way they do this *this week*? (Circle Yes/No)

        YES   NO

What is *one thing* I can do this week to engage and embrace the organization's vision and inspire others to own the vision for themselves?

_____
_____
_____
_____
_____
_____
_____
_____
_____
_____
_____

MODULE 3

Fostering Leadership

• • •

Collaborative team leadership is necessary for fluid employee communication, high colleague engagement, and empowerment.

~ Pamela Tripp

Reading Notes: Chapter 5
Use the following pages to take notes while you read. Pay special attention to concepts you think would be interesting to discuss at your MMG meeting:

_____
_____
_____
_____
_____
_____
_____
_____
_____
_____
_____
_____
_____
_____
_____
_____

The Culture Cure Mastermind Guide for Healthcare Transformation

MASTERMIND DISCUSSION GUIDE
Module 3: Fostering Leadership
Chapter 5

DISCUSSION TOPIC #1:
My ability to lead depends on my relationships—not my job title.

In chapter 5 of *The Culture Cure*, we explore the power of a workplace where everyone embraces a leadership mindset. Even if you don't have people who directly report to you, you are a leader. You have to lead yourself! Your ability to lead is not limited by your title, only your influence. Over time, when you go above and beyond and give your best to your work, people notice and your circle of influence expands.

People will not follow you if they cannot trust you; but if they trust you, they will engage with your leadership. It's not about being perfect or right all the time. It's about being the best you can be, and admitting to mistakes. Being transparent. You have to own your job and your responsibility. Lead yourself first, and become someone worth following.

I. Am I known as a team player? Do people like working with me?
___
___
___
___
___
___
___

II. How dependable am I? Do I have the characteristics of trustworthiness, excellence, and consistency? Where do I have room to grow in these areas?

_____
_____
_____
_____
_____
_____

III. Do I know what my own core values are? Am I living my core values at work?

_____
_____
_____
_____
_____
_____

II. IDEA STARTERS:

   A. **Put Yourself Out There**. Get involved, volunteer for leadership opportunities, and be engaged in the discussion and strategy opportunities whenever they arise. One of the fastest ways to get to know yourself is to step into leadership opportunities. How often do you turn down small opportunities to lead? Instead of saying no next time, say YES!
   B. **The 3:1 Approach**. Brainstorm 3 Possible Solutions for every 1 problem or challenge at work. Don't stop there! Take the possible solutions to the leader or manager who could help you make change happen. And remember: if they offer to let you lead to

implement a solution, take them up on it! This is how you grow your circle of influence.

CHALLENGE: It always seems easier to complain than to roll up your sleeves and be part of a solution. Being part of a solution to a problem grows you personally and professionally.

DISCUSSION TOPIC #2:
Prioritization of my own work is an act of leadership.

Whether you have someone reporting to you at work or not, you play a major leadership role every day. That is being CEO of your own job. The first person you lead is YOU! When you decide where to put your focus, which things to prioritize over others, you are making leadership decisions.

As joint leaders in our work, how we prioritize our work has a major impact on the organization. In *The Culture Cure* chapter 5, the 3-3-3-1 Leadership Principle is introduced. It states that to have a healthy culture we need to spend 30% of our time caring about CULTURE (colleagues and patients), 30% of our time caring about QUALITY (systems), 30% of our time caring about FINANCE (stewardship), and 10% caring about GOVERNANCE (accountability).

I. How much of the time in your organization is focused on mandatory or required governance measures? If it's more than 10% of time, what other areas are suffering?

_____
_____
_____
_____
_____
_____
_____

II. Do I make people and their well being a priority? Or does the human side take a back seat to the urgency of tasks and regulatory hoops? If I was putting people in the first 30% of my focus, what changes would I make in how I approach or execute my work on a daily basis?

_____
_____
_____
_____
_____
_____
_____

III. Do I see myself as being at the mercy of everyone else's priorities? If being a leader means OWNING my own priorities first, what changes do I need to make in my prioritization?

_____
_____
_____
_____
_____
_____
_____

II. IDEA STARTERS:

    A. **Keep it In front Of You.** Sometimes something as simple as a sticky note can be all the reminder we need. Post the following diagram where you'll see it as you make these decisions throughout the day. Put the note inside your badge, or at your desk—anywhere that will give you the reminder that YOU are the CEO of your job. And YOU make the decisions that matter!

30%	- PEOPLE	(This builds Culture.)*
30%	- SYSTEMS	(This yields Quality.)
30%	- STEWARDSHIP	(This protects Finances.)
10%	- ACCOUNTABILITY	(This satisfies Governance.)

*This is First Priority

B. **Why Bother?** The biggest barrier to creating a culture of leadership is the "why bother" mentality. Anytime we buy the untruth that our words and actions don't make a difference, we're letting our personal leadership die. So BOTHER! Every time you behave as a leader—of yourself or others—it causes a ripple effect in your work environment. If you're in a position to do so, consider establishing an **"I LEAD" Award** that can be given anytime someone steps up to care for the organization. Something as simple as an award pin, candy bar, or write-up can go a long way to reinforce leadership in the culture.

BEWARE: Most prioritization mistakes come from spending too much focus on REGULATION, asking "what do I HAVE to do in order to get or stay in compliance." Flip the paradigm and concentrate on 3.3.3.1 Leadership Principle. When your leadership and organizational priorities are in appropriate order and focus, regulatory mandates take care of themselves. Culture (people) must come first.

SELF-REFLECTION & ACTION
MODULE 3: FOSTERING LEADERSHIP
CHAPTER 5

It's all about my personal attitude and action. What am I going to do to embody and inspire others?

FOUR I'S MODEL OF SELF-REFLECTION

How can I....

❑ How can I be INSPIRED by the content that I have learned? What are ways that my colleagues and I can inspire and encourage people with these ideas?

_____
_____
_____
_____
_____
_____

❑ How can I INFLUENCE others in my behaviors based on my new awareness? How can I personally use my influence to reflect and draw these behaviors out in others?

_____
_____
_____
_____
_____
_____

❑ How can I INNOVATE among my colleagues to sustain my new learning? How can we bring innovation with this into our workplace?

_____
_____
_____
_____
_____
_____
_____

❑ How can I IMPACT my overall work environment based on my learning experience?

_____
_____
_____
_____
_____
_____
_____

FACILITATOR'S NOTE: Do not allow participants to move to the action steps without adequate time for self-reflection and processing of module material. Self-reflection is key to learning.

Take Action

Who do you know who is a great example of creating a *leadership environment*?

_____

Will you find a chance to tell them you've noticed them, and appreciate the way they lead themselves *this week*? (Circle Yes/No)

           YES   NO

What is *one thing* I can do this week to encourage a leadership environment for myself and others?

_____
_____
_____
_____
_____
_____
_____
_____
_____
_____
_____
_____
_____

MODULE 4

Engage Empathy

• • •

Possessing empathy allows a person's heart not to be self-absorbed and self-centered, it sensitizes one's heart to others.

~ Pamela Tripp

Reading Notes: Chapter 6

Use the following pages to take notes while you read. Pay special attention to concepts you think would be interesting to discuss at your MMG meeting:

_____
_____
_____
_____
_____
_____
_____
_____
_____
_____
_____
_____
_____
_____

The Culture Cure Mastermind Guide for Healthcare Transformation

Pamela M Tripp MEd, MSOM

MASTERMIND DISCUSSION GUIDE
Module 4: Regaining Empathy
Chapter 6

DISCUSSION TOPIC #1:
Empathy Deficit Disorder (EDD)

In *The Culture Cure* chapter 6, the author introduces "Empathy Deficit Disorder." This condition is often characterized by a numbness to, or difficulty understanding the feelings and perspectives of others. It is a desensitization to the experiences of others, often caused in organizations by prolonged existence in survival mode.

Not being able to feel what others are feeling creates a ripple effect in our communication, and level of caring and understanding with others. If we can't empathize with what they're experiencing, research shows that communication issues like bullying, and workplace inequality are likely to increase.

I. Do you believe there is an empathy deficit in your organization, or the world in general? Do any examples come to mind?

_____
_____
_____
_____
_____
_____
_____

II. Do you feel that YOU are experiencing an empathy deficit at home or work? How is it showing up in your words, attitudes, actions?

_____
_____
_____
_____
_____
_____
_____

III. Empathy deficit often comes because we don't take the time to get to know people. What are some things you do that may be barriers to getting to know others in a meaningful way?

_____
_____
_____
_____
_____
_____
_____

IDEA STARTERS:

A. **WATF**. To check in with your empathy, try asking yourself "**W**hat **A**re **T**hey **F**eeling?" several times a day. See how many times you can ask yourself this question when interacting with others each day! Get in the habit of asking this question for every person you interact with.

B. **Shadowing & Rounding**: If you want an advanced understanding of someone else's pressures and experience at work, ask to **Shadow** them. Do what they do, and learn their role by stepping into it with them for a while. If formal shadowing isn't available, volunteer to help them and tune your mind to imagine what it would be like to have this be your role every day.

You can also get a great deal more understanding by paying attention and valuing the perspectives of colleagues when you engage in the practice of **Rounding**. Don't dismiss the observations or concerns of colleagues who are different from you. Think about how they reached their conclusion and ask questions to deepen your empathy.

It's HUMAN to imagine we know what other people are feeling; it's SUPER HUMAN to step into their shoes to experience it ourselves.

DISCUSSION TOPIC #2:
"Survival Mode" is the archenemy of empathy.

Quite often, empathy isn't lost out of spite, but rather self-absorption. Our ability to feel for others is lost when we're preoccupied with our own worries. The way we treat people when we're focused on surviving doesn't leave room for empathy. We desire to be kind—but we just don't have time. We can't help them out—we're barely making it ourselves.

If you've ever heard someone say "I can't care about that right now," you're seeing survival mode in action. Survival mode has its benefits, but when we stay in it for too long, it threatens the culture.

I. Do you, or others on your team seem to be living in survival mode? How long has it been that way?

_____
_____
_____
_____
_____
_____
_____

II. Whose needs (other than your own) do you see going unmet? Who (outside of yourself) seems to be struggling to survive?

_____
_____
_____
_____
_____
_____
_____

III. Who have you written off at work as being uncaring, unhelpful, or rude? Are they in survival mode? Have you ever behaved in a similar way when you were stressed?

_____
_____
_____
_____
_____
_____
_____

Idea Starters:

A. **Make a Point to Celebrate.** One powerful way to pull out of survival mode is celebrating progress you've made or victories you've had. When was the last time you celebrated a victory at work (or at home!)? What recent victory has happened that you could celebrate to draw your team out of survival mode? Spend your words at work acknowledging progress, and drawing attention to victories big and small.

B. **Help Someone Else.** If your burden is feeling heavy, find one person whose burden you can lighten. Often others struggle with things that are easy for us. By allowing ourselves to care about the struggles of another person, we are telling our brains that we aren't in survival mode. It helps us switch off the survival mentality, and energizes our other work. You'll find that the energy boost you gain from giving a boost to others can be the difference maker in getting your own work done!

REMEMBER: When you're living in survival mode, the best you can hope is that you survive.

SELF-REFLECTION & ACTION
MODULE 4: REGAINING EMPATHY
CHAPTER 6

It's all about my personal attitude and action. What am I going to do to embody and inspire others?

FOUR I'S MODEL OF SELF-REFLECTION

How can I....

❏ How can I be INSPIRED by the content that I have learned? What are ways that my colleagues and I can inspire and encourage people with these ideas?

_____
_____
_____
_____
_____
_____

❏ How can I INFLUENCE others in my behaviors based on my new awareness? How can I personally use my influence to reflect and draw these behaviors out in others?

_____
_____
_____
_____
_____
_____

- How can I INNOVATE among my colleagues to sustain my new learning? How can we bring innovation with this into our workplace?

___

- How can I IMPACT my overall work environment based on my learning experience?

___

FACILITATOR'S NOTE: Do not allow participants to move to the action steps without adequate time for self-reflection and processing of module material. Self-reflection is key to learning.

Take Action

Who do you know who is a great example of demonstrating *empathy* in their attitude and actions?

_____

Will you find a chance to tell them you've noticed them, and appreciate the way they do this *this week*? (Circle Yes/No)

              YES   **NO**

What is *one thing* I can do this week to re-engage empathy for myself and others?

_____
_____
_____
_____
_____
_____
_____
_____
_____
_____
_____
_____

MODULE 5

Taking Ownership

• • •

Ownership means never hiding behind the statement "that's not my job." It is investing the best of you to get the best out of your organization.

~ Pamela Tripp

Reading Notes: Chapter 7

Use the following pages to take notes while you read. Pay special attention to concepts you think would be interesting to discuss at your MMG meeting:

_____
_____
_____
_____
_____
_____
_____
_____
_____
_____
_____
_____
_____
_____
_____
_____

The Culture Cure Mastermind Guide for Healthcare Transformation

MASTERMIND DISCUSSION GUIDE
Module 5: Taking Ownership
Chapter 7

DISCUSSION TOPIC #1:
That's Not My Job

Chapter 7 of *The Culture Cure* dives into the concept of ownership, describing ownership as a *mindset* that says you own everything—not just your job or your department. In fact, every part of the organization is yours! This means that when something goes wrong, someone needs help, or a patient has a problem; there is no room for us to say "that's not my job."

Even if something isn't your fault, choosing to own the situation—good, bad, or ugly— this gives you power. Once you own a situation, there is always something that can be done. If you have an attitude of ownership, you could be the CEO and if you see a piece of trash on the floor, you would pick it up.

I. How much ownership do you see yourself taking at work? Do you try to limit it as much as possible? What would happen if you started taking ownership of everything?

_____
_____
_____
_____
_____
_____
_____

II. The alternative to taking ownership is playing the blame game. Do you see this happening around you? What problems does this create?

_____
_____
_____
_____
_____
_____

III. When you see someone pitching in when they don't have to, what do you think of them? If someone were to take ownership of a problem they didn't create in order to find a solution, would you be more likely to listen to them when they have ideas or requests in the future?

_____
_____
_____
_____
_____
_____

IDEA STARTERS:

A. **Get Possessive.** Take pride in what your organization does daily. Use personal and team possessive words for departments other than yours. Be inclusive in thoughts and actions. It's OUR L&D department or team. They're OUR satisfaction scores. Be the person who others know can be counted on to own problems and brainstorm solutions.

B. **LEADER Buttons.** Help your teams embrace ownership by rewarding acts of ownership with a button or badge for their lanyard that says "I am a Leader".

REMEMBER: When we are characterized by saying "that's not my job," it destroys our ability to influence others.

DISCUSSION TOPIC #2:
Showing up filled up.

Have you ever heard the phrase "show up filled up?" It means looking after yourself, and doing what needs to be done so you arrive at work with a full tank of gas for the work ahead.

Taking ownership doesn't mean becoming the Lone Ranger. It means becoming the very best you can be and being determined to make a positive difference in your world. Even owning a problem doesn't mean you need to solve it alone! It means bringing your best and all of your influence to address the problem.

I. Are you taking care of yourself so that you can show up and OWN your work every day? What parts of your life are running on empty and need to be addressed?

_____
_____
_____
_____
_____
_____
_____

II. What further education or training would help you better own your work? What areas of your work leave you beyond empty after a normal work week? How could you be more sustainably "filled up?"

_____
_____
_____
_____
_____
_____
_____

III. Are there problems you're trying to fix alone? Who would you draft to give some supportive energy, ideas, or help? If you're being the Lone Ranger, stop and ask yourself, "who could help me with this?"

_____
_____
_____
_____
_____
_____

IDEA STARTERS:

A. **Adopt a Emergent Mentality.** Imagine for a moment that your team is facing a mass casualty crisis—like a highway catastrophe or weather disaster. Think for a moment about the way everyone comes together to help one another survive. Focus replaces multitasking. You don't hear people saying "that's not my job," but rather "how can I help?" We're sensitive to the fatigue of others, handing out more kudos and encouragement because we know something: everyone is exhausted but we can't quit yet. We grab sleep when we can because we know we're going to need it, and eat for fuel and focus.

   It isn't a stretch to take those realities and apply them to our everyday life. Everyone is facing stress and challenges, so let's use the spirit of "we're in this together" to become better team members.

B. **Be Your Brother's Keeper.** Sometimes along the way we can let our *independence* come to mean caring only for what happens to ourselves and not to others. Unfortunately, our workplace operates on a powerful dichotomy: no single one of us can accomplish anything of significance alone, and yet every single person has massive impact on the culture and success of the organization.

This means that when you save one person from drowning, you're really saving the organization. And when you pick up the slack someone left behind, it makes a difference to the patients and colleagues who come after you. Quit worrying about what you should and shouldn't have to do. Be the boss of you; make the difference!

REMEMBER: Taking ownership has nothing to do with blame or obligation. It's about becoming the CEO of your universe, and making the difference that you can make—simply because you can.

SELF-REFLECTION & ACTION
Module 5: Taking Ownership
Chapter 7

It's all about my personal attitude and action. What am I going to do to embody and inspire others as an individual?

Four I's Model of Self-Reflection

How can I....

- ❏ How can I be INSPIRED by the content that I have learned? What are ways that my colleagues and I inspire and encourage people with these ideas?

  _____
  _____
  _____
  _____
  _____
  _____
  _____

- ❏ How can I INFLUENCE others in my behaviors based on my new awareness? How can I personally use my influence to reflect and draw these behaviors out in others?

  _____
  _____
  _____
  _____
  _____
  _____
  _____

The Culture Cure Mastermind Guide for Healthcare Transformation

❑ How can I INNOVATE among my colleagues to sustain my new learning? How can we bring innovation with this into our workplace?

_____
_____
_____
_____
_____
_____
_____

❑ How can I IMPACT my overall work environment based on my learning experience?

_____
_____
_____
_____
_____
_____
_____

FACILITATOR'S NOTE: Do not allow participants to move to the action steps without adequate time for self-reflection and processing of module material. Self-reflection is key to learning.

Take Action

Name an individual who is a great example of a person taking ownership of their work.

_____

Be intentional about telling colleagues that you admire the way they take ownership of their job. Will you do this *this week?* (Circle Yes/No)

YES   NO

What is *one thing* I can do this week to take more ownership in my job?

Discuss what would be some benefits to an individual, their colleagues, and the organization as a whole when there is a culture of ownership?

_____
_____
_____
_____
_____
_____
_____
_____
_____
_____

MODULE 6

Developing Strengths

• • •

Leaders who value and invest in colleague's strengths will in turn develop and propel the organization to its greatest potential.

~ Pamela Tripp

Reading Notes: Chapter 8

Use the following pages to take notes while you read. Pay special attention to concepts you think would be interesting to discuss at your MMG meeting:

_____
_____
_____
_____
_____
_____
_____
_____
_____
_____
_____
_____
_____
_____
_____
_____

The Culture Cure Mastermind Guide for Healthcare Transformation

MASTERMIND DISCUSSION GUIDE
Module 6: Developing Strengths
Chapter 8

DISCUSSION TOPIC #1:
Know Your Strengths

In chapter 8 of *The Culture Cure*, we examine the value of developing the personal strengths of our healthcare colleagues. As soon as we attempt this, we will realize that many of our colleagues don't know what their strengths are. More often still, they see their own strengths through the filter of social conditioning. What were we told we were good at in school? What do our peers or employer see as strengths we "should" have?

    Often, our view of our strengths is lopsided. Perhaps we use insights from Tom Rath's famous *Strengths Finder 2.0*, which gives insights strictly in the context of work. Or we go only on what we've been told we're good at, but haven't give much thought to finding our strengths for ourselves. Today's discussion, start with you. Let's broaden your understanding of your strengths.

I. What are you personal strengths? Think beyond the *skills* you are most familiar with and think about work you like to do. When do you feel the happiness?

_____
_____
_____
_____
_____
_____
_____

II. Has someone influenced your perception of your strengths? Have you personally defined what your strengths are?

_____
_____
_____
_____
_____
_____

III. How often do you use your strengths at work? Do you feel you live in your strength zone?

_____
_____
_____
_____
_____
_____

IDEA STARTERS:

A. **Strengths In Action:** Take a new kind of strengths test at www.viacharacter.org/. This free scientific survey will help you identify your character strengths in action. Since it's a free tool, it's easy to share with colleagues to jump start their own personal strengths discovery journey.

B. **Strengths Relay:** Start a chain reaction at work. Begin the day by sharing with a colleague a strength that you see in them. Make sure you tell them *why* you value this strength to maximize the appreciation and energy boost it gives them. Begin the Strength Relay, by asking them to continue to find another colleague, and share with them a strength that they demonstrated and is valued. Add to the excitement by creating a Strengths Relay index card with each person's strength, and ask each person who gets "tagged" to sign the card and pass it on. To evaluate the strengths shared among the group, include your name and contact on the card and ask that when the card is full, to please returned to you.

REMEMBER: In order to develop our strengths, we must first KNOW and VALUE them.

DISCUSSION TOPIC #2:
The Cure For Burnout

The collective personal strengths of colleagues is the most valuable asset in any organization, impacting everything from culture to the bottom line itself. When colleagues use their strengths in daily work, they are more engaged. Conversely, when colleagues are not operating in and developing their strengths, burnout occurs.

The only way to keep people from running out of gas is to invest in helping to fill their tank. The most efficient and effective way to do that is to invest time, energy, and efforts as an organization in their personal strengths by personal and professional development.

I. How prevalent is burnout in your organization? Have you seen burnout-related turnover in your work environment?

___

II. Does your work environment show signs of work stress?

___

III. If your strengths were being utilized and developed at work, how would that better support the organization?

_____
_____
_____
_____
_____
_____
_____

IDEA STARTERS:

A. **Burnout Buster:** Anytime someone is feeling overwhelmed or stressed, a sure way to jumpstart fresh ideas and energy is to focus on their strengths. Use the self-coaching process of these three quick action steps to bust burnout. This information could be posted in staff lounges.
BURNOUT BUSTER:
1. IDENTIFY: What task or situation is making me feel tired, drained, or overwhelmed?
2. RECALL: List 2 or 3 of my personal strengths.
3. IMAGINE: How could I use one of my strengths to complete the task or address the situation that's draining.

B. **Employee Wellness Programs:** Healthcare is made up of people who are caregivers at work, and personal support to those in their personal lives as well. Finding ways to de-stress colleague environments as much as possible and instituting Employee Wellness Programs is a powerful burnout prevention strategy. Consider ways to de-institutionalize staff areas, converting staff rooms with a clinical feel to have soft lighting, comfy furniture, and creature comforts that colleagues are used to finding in their favorite cafés. Providing a non-institutional atmosphere in staff areas can provide a much-needed mental break from work. Add Wellness

Programs that offer mental health support, parenting classes, time management, financial training, and fitness and physical activities. Even short meditations at the beginning of meetings or in morning huddles are supportive to a healthy lifestyle.

What you see in people determines what you're able to draw out of them. Look for people's strengths.

SELF-REFLECTION & ACTION
MODULE 6: DEVELOPING STRENGTHS
CHAPTER 8

It's all about my personal attitude and action. What am I going to do to embody and inspire others through understanding, developing, and living out my own strengths?

FOUR I'S MODEL OF SELF-REFLECTION

How can I....

- ❏ How can I be INSPIRED by the content that I have learned? What are ways that my colleagues and I can inspire and encourage people with these ideas?

  _____
  _____
  _____
  _____
  _____
  _____

- ❏ How might I INFLUENCE others in my behaviors based on my new awareness? How can I personally use my influence to reflect and replicate similar behaviors in others?

  _____
  _____
  _____
  _____
  _____
  _____

❏ How may I INNOVATE with my colleagues to sustain my new learning? How can the innovation be used in our workplace?

_____
_____
_____
_____
_____
_____
_____

❏ What ways can I IMPACT my overall work environment based on my learning experience?

_____
_____
_____
_____
_____
_____
_____

FACILITATOR'S NOTE: Masterminds are about thought formation and reflection among a group. Do not allow participants to move to the action steps without adequate time for self-reflection and processing of module material. Self-reflection is key to learning.

Take Action

Who do you know that is a great example of *developing* their *personal strengths*?

_____

Will you find a chance to tell them you've noticed them, and appreciate the way they do this *this week*? (Circle Yes/No)

YES   NO

What is *one thing* I can do this week to develop my own personal strengths, and encourage others to do the same?

_____
_____
_____
_____
_____
_____
_____
_____
_____
_____
_____
_____

MODULE 7

Equipping Colleagues

• • •

"Equipping goes beyond the tangible tools one must possess to do their job. Equipping the human being must come first."

~ Pamela Tripp

Reading Notes: Chapter 9

Use the following pages to take notes while you read. Pay special attention to concepts you think would be interesting to discuss at your MMG meeting:

_____
_____
_____
_____
_____
_____
_____
_____
_____
_____
_____
_____
_____
_____
_____
_____

The Culture Cure Mastermind Guide for Healthcare Transformation

MASTERMIND DISCUSSION GUIDE
Module 7: Equipping Colleagues
Chapter 9

DISCUSSION TOPIC #1:
Human Needs

In chapter 9 of *The Culture Cure*, we look at a seemingly obvious, but often neglected reality: colleagues are humans first. Understanding and consistently meeting our own needs and our colleagues' human needs is paramount if we are going to create and maintain a high reliable organization.

There is a direct relationship between the success of the organization and the health and self actualization of your colleagues. The growth and development of an organization is directly proportional to the growth and development of the colleagues who work there. The purpose of understanding Maslow's Hierarchy is to cultivate a place that the human condition of colleagues is supported, so they may have place or space in which to feel a personal life quality. Use Maslow's Hierarchy depicted in this chapter to reflect on the level of the colleague's needs that you feel are being met or neglected, as it relates to your workplace environment.

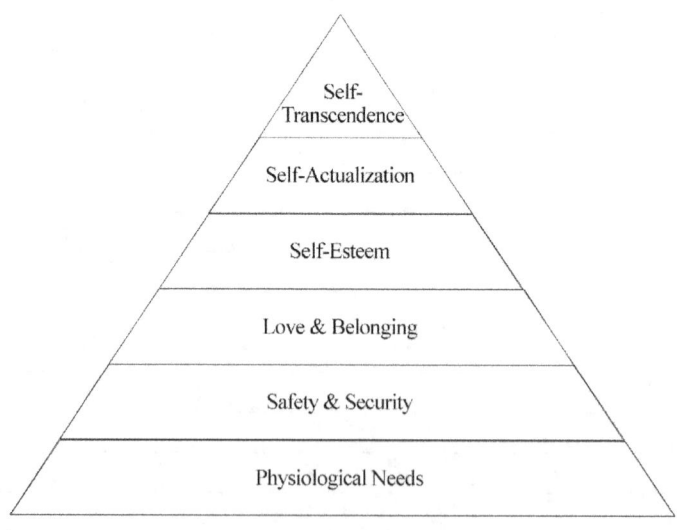

I. What level of needs do you see yourself seeking to meet? Where are your colleagues?

_____
_____
_____
_____
_____
_____

II. Do colleagues have the physical resources needed to do their jobs on a daily basis?

_____
_____
_____
_____
_____
_____

III. The ability to grow and develop ourselves is a basic human need. In what concrete ways does your organization support the Maslow Hierarchy levels of human needs?

_____
_____
_____
_____
_____
_____

IDEA STARTERS:

A. **Alter Ego Challenge:** A fun way to meet self-esteem needs is by choosing a positive alter ego to be at work. The crucial value of a strong identity can be bolstered by positive nicknames that reflect heroes or celebrities that display characteristics we share. Call yourself "the Flash" to take pride in your efforts to be quick, efficient, and meet people's needs faster than a speeding bullet. Share the love and give positive nicknames to colleagues, telling them what positive part of their identity you are basing it on.
B. **JUST ASK:** If your organization hasn't been characterized by meeting the needs of colleagues and equipping them well, it's easy to stop speaking up. Remember the insights you gained in the Ownership Module; when you need something, make it your mantra to "Just ask."

REMEMBER: We are always working at a conscious or subconscious level to meet our human needs at some level of Maslow's Hierarchy.

DISCUSSION TOPIC #2:
Creating a Learning Environment

A learning environment is one that fosters questioning and innovation. It is a safe place to evaluate what you're doing every day to see how you can improve it together. In a learning environment, we seek to improve, and transform. When these adjustments become part of the work norm, we no longer react to innovation as being a "fearful change."

I. People share thoughts and ideas in a learning environment, because it is a safe place to question. How safe is your work environment for questions? When you have a new idea to improve your work performance or the organization's operational work, do you share it? If so how and to whom?

_____
_____
_____
_____
_____
_____

II. How do YOU respond when others share new ideas about work improvements?

_____
_____
_____
_____
_____
_____
_____

III. In what meaningful ways do you feel your organization would benefit from being a learning environment of creativity and innovation?

_____
_____
_____
_____
_____
_____
_____

IDEA STARTERS:

A. **Start a Culture Council:** Form and charter a culture transformation council, consisting of a cross-section of the your organization to innovate ways to improve the culture in your organization. This special team provides oversight for cultural excellence. Members of the council are the "Eagles" in your organization who represent colleagues and leaders. An informal start could come in the form of focus groups, tasked to improve specific elements of work culture, patient care, or team processes.

B. **Newsletter Spotlight:** Spotlight people who ask questions and/or have innovative ideas in the organization's newsletter. Tell their story and praise them in print for reinforcement of a learning culture. By drawing positive attention to questions and innovation it sends the message that your organization is ready to make things better, and will listen when colleagues voice ideas. Make it official and announce something like **"The Ingenuity Award,"** given to the individual or team who shows stellar critical thinking, asks the hard questions, and comes up with ingenious innovation.

REMEMBER: In a learning environment, it doesn't matter where a good idea comes from.

SELF-REFLECTION & ACTION
Module 7: Equipping Colleagues
Chapter 9

It's all about my personal attitude and action. What am I going to do to embody and inspire others?

Four I's Model of Self-Reflection

How can I….

❏ How can I be INSPIRED by the content that I have learned? What are ways that my colleagues and I can inspire and encourage people with these ideas?

_____
_____
_____
_____
_____
_____
_____

❏ How can I INFLUENCE others in my behaviors based on my new awareness? How can I personally use my influence to reflect and draw these behaviors out in others?

_____
_____
_____
_____
_____
_____
_____

❏ How can I INNOVATE among my colleagues to sustain a learning environment? How can we bring innovation with this into our workplace?

_____
_____
_____
_____
_____
_____
_____

❏ How can I IMPACT my overall work environment based on my learning experience?

_____
_____
_____
_____
_____
_____
_____

FACILITATOR'S NOTE: Do not allow participants to move to the action steps without adequate time for self-reflection and processing of module material. Self-reflection is key to learning.

Take Action

Who do you know who is a great example of *equipping colleagues*?

_____

Will you find a chance to tell them you've noticed them, and appreciate the way they do this *this week*? (Circle Yes/No)

          YES   **NO**

What is *one thing* I can do this week to be equipped, and encourage others to do the same?

_____
_____
_____
_____
_____
_____
_____
_____
_____
_____
_____
_____
_____
_____

MODULE 8

Unleashing Empowerment

• • •

"Develop colleagues' strengths, and colleague empowerment will become the expected evolution of excellence in your work environment."

~ Pamela Tripp

Reading Notes: Chapter 10

Use the following pages to take notes while you read. Pay special attention to concepts you think would be interesting to discuss at your MMG meeting:

_____
_____
_____
_____
_____
_____
_____
_____
_____
_____
_____
_____
_____
_____
_____
_____

The Culture Cure Mastermind Guide for Healthcare Transformation

MASTERMIND DISCUSSION GUIDE
Module 8: Unleashing Empowerment
Chapter 10

DISCUSSION TOPIC #1:
Set Up To Fail

In chapter 10 of *The Culture Cure* we explore empowerment. Empowerment unleashes excellence on a broad scale by effectively sharing power and authority. We never empower someone without ensuring that we have equipped them first. We must nourish people's knowledge, performance levels, and skill sets to ensure success and not a set up for failure.

Empowerment also has to be accompanied with forgiveness. Punitive environments are not empowerment environments. Leaders who desire to unleash the power of their people, are continually finding ways of equipping them first. Leaders should also anticipate the natural learning curve, and the minor bumps that growth of colleagues will have along the way. The result of an empowering environment is a major improvement being unleashed in the culture, quality of care, financial success, and regulatory compliance in your organization.

I. Discuss opportunities for empowerment to be practiced more in your organization. What initial steps should be taken to achieve this?

_____
_____
_____
_____
_____
_____
_____

II. Are colleagues effectively equipped to handle the responsibilities they are given in your organization? How can the lack of equipping undermine the value of empowering colleagues?

_____
_____
_____
_____
_____
_____

III. What does the concept of "forgiveness" mean to you in the context of empowering colleagues? What is the behavior expected around a colleague's "mistake" in an organization of growth?

_____
_____
_____
_____
_____
_____

IDEA STARTERS:

A. **#SoThatHappened:** An empowered culture is one that handles the unexpected (including colleague mistakes) without becoming hostile. When something goes wrong, take a pause, and use that time to self reflect and learn. Was better equipping of the colleague needed? This pause helps to diffuse the unnecessary emotional pressure created by the unexpected event, and gives your brain time to catch up with possible solutions.

B. **Best Learning Opportunity:** Take the shame out of mistakes by actually rewarding colleagues who embrace their empowerment and find things less than perfect. Taking the time to acknowledge the thought process and bravery to attempt solving problems—even in situations where everything doesn't work out perfectly—teaches colleagues to value critical thinking, self-reflection, and willingness to try to improve things.

REMEMBER: No single leader can do everything. Empowerment multiplies leadership.

DISCUSSION TOPIC #2:
Micromanagement Is Not Leadership

Insecure leaders struggle with empowerment of others. Instead of empowering, they exert excessive control. "Just do as I say," is a micromanagement mode. This kind of control creates a major leadership lid, limiting the power of the leader and capacity for team performance. Things like seeking input, delegating decision making, and not having to have the final word are all elements of a collaborative leadership model. At the end of the day, empowerment is sharing power. Strong leaders develop their influence, not their control.

I. Do you micromanage? Do you observe micromanagement in your organization? How do you feel when you are micromanaged?

_____
_____
_____
_____
_____
_____
_____

II. Discuss times that you have participated in the micromanagement of others. What did you learn from the experience?

_____
_____
_____
_____
_____
_____
_____

III. How can you begin collaboration and sharing your power with others?

_____
_____
_____
_____
_____
_____
_____

IDEA STARTERS:

A. **No Yo-Yo:** Sometimes a leader may practice empowerment one day, and then takes back control. This type of yo-yo leadership kills trust and de-energizes the team. Think about opportunities such as new projects, that requires a team to complete. Intentionally design the team charter to support collaborative responsibilities assigned. Recognize the contribution of each individual to the team's success.

B. **MACRO-Manager Award:** Make a point to give a "Macromanager Award" to colleagues who resist the temptation of micromanaging in their department. Equipping and then empowering colleagues is brave leadership, so give kudos where kudos is due!

KEY REALITY: Continuous equipping makes it possible to continuously empower colleagues. Don't give responsibility without preparing the colleague to succeed.

SELF-REFLECTION & ACTION
Module 8: Unleashing Empowerment
Chapter 10

It's all about my personal attitude and action. What can I do to embody and inspire others?

Four I's Model of Self-Reflection

How can I....

- ❏ How can I be INSPIRED by the content that I have learned? What are ways that my colleagues and I can inspire and encourage people?

  _____
  _____
  _____
  _____
  _____
  _____

- ❏ How can I INFLUENCE others in my behaviors based on my new awareness? How can I personally use my influence to reflect and draw these behaviors out in others?

  _____
  _____
  _____
  _____
  _____
  _____

- ❏ How can I INNOVATE among my colleagues to sustain my new learning model? How can I bring innovation into my workplace?

  _____
  _____
  _____
  _____
  _____
  _____
  _____

- ❏ How can I IMPACT my overall work environment based on my learning experience?

  _____
  _____
  _____
  _____
  _____
  _____
  _____

FACILITATOR'S NOTE: Do not allow participants to move to the action steps without adequate time for self-reflection and processing of module material. Self-reflection is key to learning.

Take Action

What actions in your environment is a great example of *empowering colleagues*?

_____

Will you find a chance to tell them you've noticed them, and appreciate the way they do this *this week*? (Circle Yes/No)

                  YES   **NO**

What is *one thing* I can do this week to empower others, and encourage others to do the same?

_____
_____
_____
_____
_____
_____
_____
_____
_____
_____
_____
_____

MODULE 9

Driving Momentum

• • •

"Momentum is a synergistic value from your greatest resource—people."

~ Pamela Tripp

Reading Notes: Chapter 11

Use the following pages to take notes while you read. Pay special attention to concepts you think would be interesting to discuss at your MMG meeting:

_____
_____
_____
_____
_____
_____
_____
_____
_____
_____
_____
_____
_____
_____
_____
_____
_____

The Culture Cure Mastermind Guide for Healthcare Transformation

MASTERMIND DISCUSSION GUIDE
Module 9: Driving Momentum
Chapter 11

DISCUSSION TOPIC #1:
Where Momentum Happens

Momentum is the collective energy force of an organization, built over time among colleagues. Surges in momentum can reach a massive scale because of the connectedness and engagement of colleagues. In fact, peers influence one another more than leaders do in many ways. That peer-to-peer energy is the largest generator and amplifier of momentum.

Begin by assessing momentum in your organization. Use the information in chapter 11 of *The Culture Cure* to see where your organization is at. Note that being stuck in the *status quo* thwarts momentum. Innovation is the springboard for building new momentum!

I. How would you describe your organization's momentum? Is it currently in low, medium, or high momentum state? Why?

_____
_____
_____
_____
_____
_____
_____

II. Do you sense peer-to-peer momentum moving the organization? Is this in a positive or negative direction?

_____
_____
_____
_____
_____
_____
_____

III. How attached is your organization to keeping things status quo? Where do you see room for improvement?

_____
_____
_____
_____
_____
_____
_____

IDEA STARTERS:

A. **Recognize Positive Action:** Momentum building is intentional and constant. It requires constant assessment by leadership. Ask for suggestions from peers on way the organization can support positive energy within the organization.

B. **Investment Inventory:** Look for ways to increase the investment value of your colleagues. This a internal personal development as depicted in the author's Corporate Transcendence™ curriculum.

REMEMBER: Building momentum takes time. Invest in colleagues to generate momentum that lasts.

DISCUSSION TOPIC #2:
Momentum Makers & Breakers

Refer to the list of "Momentum Drainers" (page 147) and "Momentum Builders" (page 148) in chapter 11 of *The Culture Cure*. Things like distrust, negativity, and unresolved conflict are just a few things that characterize a low momentum organization. Active empathy, effective workflow, and transparency are a few things present in high momentum organizations.

I. What Momentum Drainers are prevalent in your organization? How do you see them impacting your ability to build momentum?

_____
_____
_____
_____
_____
_____
_____

II. What Momentum Builders do you see in your organization? Noticing positive signs is crucial for building the momentum you want.

_____
_____
_____
_____
_____
_____
_____

III. If you were to pick one Momentum Drainer you'd most like to get rid of in your work culture, and one Momentum Builder you want most to increase, what would they be?

_____
_____
_____
_____
_____
_____
_____

IDEA STARTERS:

A. **Reward and Recognition:** Improvements and success in organizations build momentum. Develop a Reward and Recognition Team that works with leaders to recognize internal and external achievements for the organization.
B. **Colleague Appreciation Day or Week:** Develop a team to create a colleague appreciation day or week. Simple things like cookies, popcorn, or small gifts can be given. It is a dedicated time to say "thank you" for their many efforts for keeping the positive progression of the organization on course.

REMEMBER: Leaders and colleagues alike make or break momentum on a daily basis.

SELF-REFLECTION & ACTION
Module 9: Driving Momentum
Chapter 11

It's all about my personal attitude and action. What am I going to do to embody and inspire others?

Four I's Model of Self-Reflection

How can I....

- ❏ How can I be INSPIRED by the content that I have learned? What are ways that my colleagues and I can inspire and encourage people with these ideas?

  _____
  _____
  _____
  _____
  _____
  _____
  _____

- ❏ How can I INFLUENCE others in my behaviors based on my new awareness? How can I personally use my influence to reflect and draw these behaviors out in others?

  _____
  _____
  _____
  _____
  _____
  _____
  _____

❏ How can I INNOVATE among my colleagues to sustain my new learning? How can we bring innovation with this into our workplace?

_____
_____
_____
_____
_____
_____
_____

❏ How can I IMPACT my overall work environment based on my learning experience?

_____
_____
_____
_____
_____
_____
_____

FACILITATOR'S NOTE: Do not allow participants to move to the action steps without adequate time for self-reflection and processing of module material. Self-reflection is key to learning.

Take Action

Who do you know who is a great example of *driving momentum*, and contributing to Momentum Builders?

_____

Will you find a chance to tell them you've noticed them, and appreciate the way they do this *this week*? (Circle Yes/No)

YES   NO

What is *one thing* I can do this week to drive momentum, and encourage others to do the same?

_____
_____
_____
_____
_____
_____
_____
_____
_____
_____
_____
_____
_____

MODULE 10

Hardwiring Success

• • •

"A silver bullet for success does not exist. Success is found in the moment-to-moment actions that people take collectively to hardwire excellence."

~ Pamela Tripp

Reading Notes: Chapter 12

Use the following pages to take notes while you read. Pay special attention to concepts you think would be interesting to discuss at your MMG meeting:

_____
_____
_____
_____
_____
_____
_____
_____
_____
_____
_____
_____
_____
_____
_____

The Culture Cure Mastermind Guide for Healthcare Transformation

Pamela M Tripp MEd, MSOM

MASTERMIND DISCUSSION GUIDE
Module 10: Hardwiring Success
Chapter 12

DISCUSSION TOPIC #1:
Defining Success

In chapter 12 of *The Culture Cure*, the entire culture transformation process comes full circle. We know and declare our organizations as being truly successful when our patients are healthier by tracking their health outcomes. We ultimately define success in terms of how well we care for our patients. This describes not only success but significance. We change our patient's lives by influencing our colleagues or our caregivers lives. The only way to have a high reliable organization with consistent, excellent patient outcomes, is to start by caring for the employee's needs, continually developing them, and elevating the work done every day.

When we take this path to success, both the patient and the colleague enjoy the fruit of success every day in the organization. Definitions of success that begin and end with financial solvency or governmental compliance create organizations that struggle, burn out colleagues, and ultimately fail. To save our patients we must put the oxygen mask on our colleagues, so they can place it on the patient.

I. How does your organization define success? How much emphasis is placed on patient outcomes? How much is placed on colleague engagement?

_____
_____
_____
_____
_____
_____

II. What is *your* definition of success at work, for yourself and the organization where you work?

_____
_____
_____
_____
_____
_____
_____

III. Siloes thwart the consistent delivery of high quality patient outcomes. Does your organization have departmental silos? What can be done in your organization to build better relationships?

_____
_____
_____
_____
_____
_____
_____

IDEA STARTERS:

A. **Word Search:** When we asked people what words best described the American healthcare system, they used words like chaotic, siloed, stressed, burnout, and even deadly. What are the words people may use to describe YOUR healthcare organization?

Get a fresh picture of how your specific organization is by asking colleagues to share with you 3 words that describe their experience in their work culture. To see how your organization progresses, repeat the word search once a quarter. Are their any changes? To help the team visualize the culture, create a word cloud using a free online word cloud tool, and post it in an employee area.

B. **A Full Picture:** Measuring the excellence of your culture should include efforts to evaluate all sectors: patient outcomes, financial viability, governance compliance, and the culture itself. If your success evaluation tools overlook the vital element of culture, conduct a simple survey, asking everyone to finish the statement: "My ideal would culture would be_____."

FACT: High reliable organizations achieve their financial success because they define success in terms of the people giving and receiving care.

DISCUSSION TOPIC #2:
The Oxygen Mask Principle

The Oxygen Mask Principle says that if we are going to heal the sickness in our healthcare organizations, we have to start by giving life-preserving care to the healthcare colleague before we can care for the patient. When we care for colleagues first, connecting them to their strengths and to one another by removing silos and developing an integrated health team, we have the recipe for a successful high reliable healthcare organization.

I. Do you agree with the author that healthcare is best healed from the inside? Why or why not?

_____
_____
_____
_____
_____
_____
_____

II. Have you seen the effects of violating the Oxygen Mask Principle? What happens when chronically drained, under-resourced colleagues care for patients?

_____
_____
_____
_____
_____
_____
_____

III. What is one thing that the organization could do to care for its colleagues better? Which leaders could you discuss this idea with in hopes of improving the strength of the colleagues at your organization?

_____
_____
_____
_____
_____
_____
_____

IDEA STARTERS:

A. **Thank You:** Create a THANK YOU Culture in your organization be truly embracing the power of gratitude. Something as simple as saying thank you *every time* you interact with another colleague creates a connection of shared positive emotion among colleagues. Gratitude is the quickest and easiest way to create shared positive emotion, which is the fuel every colleague needs in order to operate at their best. People need regular doses of this shared positive emotion in order to create a high reliable organization where patients get the best care.

B. **6 Foot Rule:** Make it a team rule to SMILE and ACKNOWLEDGE every human who gets within 6 feet of you. Not just once a day, but every time someone enters your 6 foot radius, give eye contact and smile. This practice lifts the spirits of colleagues and values them as people. Try it this week!

REMEMBER: Healthcare colleagues are humans first. Successful organizations thrive because they create teams of healthy humans helping humans become healthy.

SELF-REFLECTION & ACTION
MODULE 10: HARDWIRING SUCCESS
CHAPTER 12

It's all about my personal attitude and action. What am I going to do to embody and inspire others?

FOUR I'S MODEL OF SELF-REFLECTION

How can I....

- ❏ How can I be INSPIRED by the content that I have learned? What are ways that my colleagues and I can inspire and encourage people with these ideas?

  _____
  _____
  _____
  _____
  _____
  _____

- ❏ How can I INFLUENCE others in my behaviors based on my new awareness? How can I personally use my influence to reflect and draw these behaviors out in others?

  _____
  _____
  _____
  _____
  _____
  _____

❏ How can I INNOVATE among my colleagues to sustain my new learning? How can we bring innovation with this into our workplace?

_____
_____
_____
_____
_____
_____
_____

❏ How can I IMPACT my overall work environment based on my learning experience?

_____
_____
_____
_____
_____
_____
_____

FACILITATOR'S NOTE: Do not allow participants to move to the action steps without adequate time for self-reflection and processing of module material. Self-reflection is key to learning.

Take Action

Who do you know who is hardwiring success by *defining success well* and *honoring the Oxygen Mask Principle*?

_____

Will you find a chance to tell them you've noticed them, and appreciate the way they do this *this week*? (Circle Yes/No)

           YES   NO

What is *one thing* I can do this week to hardwire success, and encourage others to do the same?

_____
_____
_____
_____
_____
_____
_____
_____
_____
_____
_____
_____

About the Author

• • •

Pamela M. Tripp, MEd, MSOM—Founder and President of Corporate Transcendence™—is a passionate culture expert, author, speaker, seasoned healthcare leader, and mentor with the John Maxwell Team. Investing over 24 years of practical research, Pamela has developed Corporate Transcendence™, a transformational curriculum for organizational excellence that guarantees sustainable success in critical areas of Culture, Quality, Finance, and Governance.

Pamela has fully tested her curriculum on the ground level and successfully taken an organization with debilitating debt and major operational problems, to become a solvent, sustainable health system, winning over 36 state and national service excellence awards—including Malcolm Baldrige Governor's Award and the Most Outstanding Healthcare Organization by the National Rural Health Association. Pamela is author of, *The Culture Cure: Transforming the Modern Healthcare System*, and its companion, *The Culture Cure Mastermind Guide for Healthcare Transformation*.

The Culture Cure shares discoveries as a senior leader and culturist in healthcare to reframe today's healthcare organizations for transformational excellence. Ms. Tripp has received national recognitions and awards for her leadership and passion to transform healthcare in America. Most recently she was honored with the NC Blue Cross Blue Shield Robert J. Gretyzn Jr. Award for Healthcare Leadership Excellence. Ms. Tripp's passion is to partner with healthcare leaders, so the American healthcare industry will be recognized as the premier model of healthcare for the world.

Learn more about Pamela at www.PamelaTripp.com and follow her on social media for ongoing insights and encouragement from the frontlines of healthcare transformation in the United States of America.

Corporate Transcendence

• • •

Is Your Organization Experiencing...

- ➤ Leadership Management Burn Out?
- ➤ High Employee Turn Over?
- ➤ Low Employee Engagement?
- ➤ Lack of Team Cohesiveness?
- ➤ Disappointing Patient Outcomes?
- ➤ Challenged Financial Benchmarks?
- ➤ Patient and Provider Dissatisfaction?

Is Corporate Transcendence for You?

Corporate Transcendence is the culture transformation provider of choice for any organization with a vision to become a high reliable integrated health care organization. Proven to heal organizations deemed beyond repair, the Corporate Transcendence Curriculum can be counted on to take any organization on a direct journey to award-winning excellence in patient care.

Corporate Transcendence provides an intentional blueprint that engages all employees within every department of your organization. If your organization isn't living up to its potential, consistently struggling to meet necessary benchmarks, Corporate Transcendence can change the trend and set a new course for excellence.

Stop wasting time, energy, and resources, into programs that fizzle. Corporate Transcendence will transform your organization from a stressed, siloed, disengaged work environment, into a growth-oriented learning environment that meets patient-centered, value-based healthcare needs of today! Become the organization of excellence you deserve to be! **Start Your Culture Transformation Today at www.CorporateTranscendence.com.**

www.ingramcontent.com/pod-product-compliance
Lightning Source LLC
Chambersburg PA
CBHW050104230526
45470CB00004B/1667